# When Time Runs Out

*Navigating Fertility in a World That Delays Motherhood*

By

## Adeola Olunloyo

# Copyright

**Copyright © 2024 Adeola Olunloyo**
All rights reserved.

No part of this book may be reproduced, stored in a retrieval system, or transmitted in any form or by any means, electronic, mechanical, photocopying, recording, or otherwise, without prior written permission from the publisher, except for the use of brief quotations in a book review or scholarly journal.

**For information regarding permission requests, please write to:**
fertilitycliques@gmail.com

**Disclaimer:**
The information contained in this book is intended for educational purposes only and is not a substitute for professional medical advice, diagnosis, or treatment. Always seek the advice of your physician or other qualified health provider with any questions you may have regarding a medical condition.

# DEDICATION

I dedicate this book to all mothers without children.

The world will be incomplete without your light, love and unique gifts to humanity.

# TABLE OF CONTENTS

# WHY I WROTE THIS BOOK

*When Time Runs Out: Navigating Fertility in a World that Delays Motherhood* is more than just a book; it's a reflection of my deeply personal journey and a heartfelt call to action.

My fertility journey began when I was 42 years old. By then, I was single, independent, and had built a successful career. Despite this, I found myself navigating a painful and challenging path, grappling with fibroids, adenomyosis, and the desire to have a child. I underwent three IVF cycles, each one ending in heartbreak. The main challenge? My age. My eggs were not viable.

The emotional toll of these failed attempts was profound. It wasn't just about the physical pain—it was the mental anguish of realizing that I had waited too long. What made it even harder to bear was the knowledge that, despite my years of experience in sexual and reproductive health, I hadn't truly understood how critical timing was for fertility. I had assumed that with my education, independence, and access to healthcare, motherhood would be a given whenever I was ready.

But reality doesn't align with societal pressure that tell women "Go, get married" at all cost without context or consideration for the peculiar challenges causing the delay. For too long, we've been fed a narrative that delays essential conversations about fertility. The result? Women like me—empowered, educated, yet unprepared for the limits of biology—are left facing the harsh consequences of time running out.

Through my journey, and in conversations with fertility experts and women facing similar struggles, I came to see glaring gaps in our systems. Fertility education is often inaccessible, shrouded in stigma, or simply dismissed as a conversation for later. Meanwhile, societal norms discourage women from making proactive reproductive choices, leaving many to navigate these challenges alone and uninformed.

This book is my attempt to change that. *When Time Runs Out* is a wake-up call to every woman—and to the communities, governments, and healthcare systems that shape our decisions. It is a plea for women to reclaim their reproductive autonomy and understand the finite nature of fertility. It is a call to challenge outdated norms, dismantle the stigma surrounding fertility issues, and push for accessible, equitable fertility education and care.

I wrote this book to spark conversations that matter, to advocate for change, and to provide women with the tools and knowledge they need to make timely, empowered reproductive choices. Fertility is finite, and the decisions we make—or don't make—today can profoundly shape our futures.

To every woman reading this: you deserve to know your options. You deserve to plan your journey on your terms. And most importantly, you deserve a world that supports your choices before time runs out.

Rooting for you with love.

# INTRODUCTION: A SILENT STRUGGLE

Fertility has long been a subject cloaked in silence and misunderstanding, quietly lurking in the background of women's lives, often unnoticed until it becomes a concern. Our modern world, with its promises of endless possibility and choice, subtly assures us that time is on our side. We're encouraged to pursue education, careers, and personal growth—prioritizing independence and ambition, all under the assumption that motherhood will simply "happen" when the time is right. But for countless women, this journey toward motherhood has taken on an unexpected layer of complexity, where science, society, and self collide.

## Overview of the Changing Trends

In recent decades, we have seen a marked shift in how women approach marriage and family. Increasingly, women are prioritizing higher education, advancing in their careers, and exploring personal fulfillment before choosing to settle down and start a family. It's no wonder that, in many ways, this trend mirrors a hard-won freedom from older societal norms, offering women the chance to carve out their own timelines. However, amid these shifting values and extended timelines lies a stark biological reality: the age-related decline in fertility.

In the early 20th century, the median age for a woman's first marriage was 21, and motherhood often followed soon after. But today, the average age for first-time mothers in many developed countries has risen to the early 30s, with many women waiting even longer. Between 1970 and 2018, the proportion of women aged 35 and older who became mothers quadrupled, underscoring a drastic societal shift. On the other hand, in Sub-Saharan Africa, average age of first-time mothers is 20 years. However, there is an increasing population of women delaying childbirth till their 30s and 40s.

With this delay, however, comes a paradox: while women are achieving unprecedented heights in education, career, and financial independence, the biological window for childbearing remains inflexible. The reality is that female fertility begins to decline around age 30 and more sharply after 35, leaving many women facing an unexpected challenge in their mid-to-late thirties and beyond.

Although science and medicine offer some support through fertility treatments, assisted reproductive technologies, and egg freezing, these options cannot fully counteract the natural decline of fertility with age. Herein lies the irony—a generation of women has unprecedented control over many aspects of their lives, yet the biological clock ticks forward without pause, often catching many by surprise.

## Why This Book Matters

This book is a call to action. It's an invitation for women to confront, understand, and embrace their fertility journeys with awareness and agency. Fertility is not a topic we need to shy away from until it becomes a problem; instead, it's one we should approach with a sense of curiosity and empowerment, equipping ourselves with knowledge that can guide us toward the outcomes we desire.

While advances in reproductive technology have indeed expanded options, fertility remains a deeply personal journey with layers of societal, cultural, and emotional dimensions. For each woman, this journey is unique, influenced by values, aspirations, and circumstances. But the hope is that by understanding the realities of reproductive health—by dispelling myths, revealing truths, and navigating through the fog of societal expectations—women can make decisions about their futures that are aligned with their individual dreams, not the shifting tides of culture or the demands of the modern world.

In this book, we will explore the intersection of biology and choice, of ambition and timing. We'll draw from scientific research, personal stories, and expert insights to shed light on what it means to take charge of one's fertility in an era where timing, more than ever, feels critical. For anyone navigating this journey, consider this book a trusted companion—a source of knowledge, support, and encouragement as you chart a path toward motherhood that honors both your dreams and your biological reality.

In short, "When Time Runs Out" isn't just a guide—it's a call for each of us to pause, listen, and truly understand our bodies and our choices. This is your journey, and it begins with awareness, empowerment, and, above all, self-compassion.

# CHAPTER 1

## THE GROWING POPULATION OF SINGLE WOMEN

In a world of evolving norms, more and more women are embracing singlehood well into their 30s and 40s. What was once seen as unconventional, or even risky, is now commonplace, reflecting a society that's rapidly changing its views on relationships, marriage, and the value of independence. As women forge new paths toward autonomy and personal fulfillment, many find themselves re-evaluating traditional timelines for marriage and family—sometimes delaying them indefinitely.

### What's Causing the Delay?

Several key factors drive this growing trend, each one interwoven with the modern woman's quest for autonomy and fulfillment.

## Career Ambitions and Financial Independence

Today, career ambitions and financial goals have become powerful motivators for women. In decades past, it was not unusual for a woman's primary social role to be defined by marriage and family. But now, with access to higher education and a wider array of career paths, many women prioritize building careers before considering long-term partnerships. This shift isn't merely about achieving financial security; it's about the desire for self-definition, accomplishment, and freedom to make independent life choices.

For many women, career is deeply intertwined with personal identity. The fulfillment derived from a career can contribute to a strong sense of self, a crucial foundation for any future relationship. But with ambition comes a trade-off: the energy, time, and commitment that careers demand often mean that marriage and family are postponed until professional goals are well established. As more women realize that they can take care of themselves financially, the urgency to rely on marriage for economic stability has diminished, allowing them to approach partnerships as a matter of personal choice, not necessity.

## Personal Freedom and the Changing Dynamics of Relationships

Personal freedom is another powerful driver. Many women today embrace the opportunity to live independently, travel, explore their interests, and pursue life experiences without needing to prioritize a partner. There's a deep sense of value in getting to know oneself fully before making a lifelong commitment. Furthermore, the modern world celebrates individualism—encouraging people to be whole and fulfilled on their own, in ways that were not always embraced by past generations.

Relationships themselves have also evolved. Women and men today expect deeper connections, emotional intimacy, and shared values from partners, placing a greater emphasis on compatibility and alignment. This evolution has raised the standard for relationships, making people more discerning in choosing a partner and more cautious of entering serious commitments prematurely.

## The Cultural Shift: Modern Dating Trends, Longer Educational Paths, and Economic Challenges

Dating, too, has changed dramatically with the rise of digital platforms, social media, and a more transient, globally connected world. Online dating has made meeting people easier but often more complex, with seemingly endless options fostering what some call the "paradox of choice." Many people report feeling overwhelmed by the sheer volume of potential partners, leading to indecision, uncertainty, and, in some cases, an extended period of dating before settling down.

Additionally, extended education has become the norm. More women are pursuing advanced degrees, which can add years to their educational journeys. This, combined with student loan debt and a challenging job market, creates economic pressures that may make women less inclined to prioritize marriage and family until they feel financially secure.

Rising living costs, stagnant wages, and housing affordability are further barriers. In many urban centers, securing a stable career and financial foundation can take until one's 30s or even 40s. In this economic landscape, marriage and children may feel like goals for a distant future rather than immediate priorities.

## Statistical Trends: A Growing Population of Single Women in Their 30s and 40s

The numbers illustrate this shift strikingly. According to the U.S. Census Bureau, the proportion of women marrying by age 30 has declined significantly over the past half-century. In the 1970s, nearly 90% of women were married by age 30, but that number has dropped to roughly 50% today. Similarly, the median age of first marriage for women has increased from around 21 in 1960 to nearly 29 as of recent years.

This phenomenon extends beyond marriage to parenthood as well. Data from the Centers for Disease Control and Prevention (CDC) shows that first births among women aged 30–39 have sharply increased, while birth rates among women in their 20s have declined. From 2000 to 2020, the number of first-time mothers aged 35 and older more than doubled, reflecting a profound societal shift toward later family planning.

Globally, the trend is similar. In countries like Japan, Germany, and Italy, the average age of marriage and parenthood has risen, mirroring a universal trend of women choosing independence and career over early family formation. In fact, some estimates suggest that in several developed nations, close to a third of women in their late 30s are single.

This chapter aims to highlight these underlying trends, not as a cautionary tale, but as a reflection of the myriad choices women have today. More than ever, society is redefining the trajectory of womanhood, challenging assumptions about marriage, motherhood, and fulfillment. In the pages that follow, we'll explore how these choices are reshaping the fertility landscape and what this means for the future, offering insight into both the freedoms and the dilemmas that come with forging one's path in a world that continues to evolve.

# CHAPTER 2

## THE BIOLOGICAL REALITY OF FERTILITY

Amid the cultural transformations that have redefined relationships, careers, and life trajectories, biology remains an unyielding anchor—a reality that shapes our reproductive possibilities in ways that cannot always be deferred or manipulated. For women, the "fertility window" is a stark reminder that, no matter how much society advances, our biological clocks continue to tick to their own ancient rhythm. In this chapter, we'll explore the fundamentals of reproductive biology and dismantle common misconceptions, providing a foundation of knowledge essential to navigating fertility with clarity and realism.

### The Fertility Window

Human fertility is governed by nature's own timeline, and while men and women each have biological cycles, the duration and flexibility of these cycles differ profoundly. Women are born with a finite supply of eggs, known as oocytes, housed within their ovaries. From the onset of puberty to menopause, the number and quality of these eggs gradually decline, diminishing a woman's fertility as she ages. Generally, female fertility begins to decline noticeably after the age of 30, accelerating after age 35 and dropping steeply in the early 40s. By age 45, most women face significant challenges in conceiving naturally.

The biological mechanics of this are complex but fundamentally straightforward: the ovaries release an egg each month during ovulation, a process repeated until menopause when the egg supply is exhausted. However, as women age, both the number of remaining eggs and their quality diminish. This decline in egg quality contributes to a greater likelihood of chromosomal abnormalities, which can lead to complications such as miscarriage, failed implantation, or developmental disorders in the fetus.

In contrast, men experience a more prolonged fertility window. While male fertility does decline gradually with age—sperm quality and motility can decrease, and risks of genetic mutations increase—their bodies continuously produce sperm throughout their lives. This biological difference is why men can often father children well into their later years, while women's fertility is constrained by a far shorter timeframe. For women, nature's design offers a finite window of peak fertility that becomes less forgiving with each passing year.

## Men vs. Women: Understanding the Disparity in Fertility Timelines

The disparity in fertility timelines between men and women is one of biology's enduring realities. This difference traces back to evolutionary biology: for a woman, pregnancy represents a significant physiological investment. Once an egg is fertilized, her body is responsible for nurturing and carrying a child to term, an energy-intensive process that has shaped how female fertility evolved.

Having a finite number of high-quality eggs ensures that reproduction happens when the woman is at an age where her body is most capable of successfully supporting a pregnancy.

Men, on the other hand, can produce sperm continuously from puberty onwards, with sperm production declining in quality gradually over time but remaining viable far longer. The evolutionary perspective here suggests that because sperm production requires far less energy and physical commitment than pregnancy, men can afford a more extended reproductive lifespan.

But while men's fertility does have longevity, it is not immune to the effects of aging. Studies show that as men age, sperm quality can decline, leading to increased risks of DNA fragmentation and genetic mutations. Advanced paternal age has been linked to higher risks of certain genetic conditions, such as autism spectrum disorders and schizophrenia. Nevertheless, while advanced paternal age can introduce reproductive challenges, it seldom poses the same abrupt biological cutoff that women face with menopause.

## The Misconceptions: Unpacking Common Myths About Women's Fertility

In today's world, reproductive technology has ushered in a sense of optimism that fertility challenges can be solved with medical intervention, giving rise to misconceptions that sometimes cloud women's understanding of their reproductive timelines. However, treatments like in vitro fertilization (IVF) and egg freezing, while revolutionary, are not guarantees—they are tools that come with limitations.

## IVF as a Guarantee of Pregnancy Success

In vitro fertilization has been a transformative development in reproductive medicine, enabling millions of people to conceive who otherwise might not have been able to. However, the success rate of IVF declines significantly as women age, precisely because egg quality diminishes with time. For women under 35, IVF has a success rate of around 40% per cycle, but by age 40, that rate falls to approximately 20%, and by 44, it drops to around 5%. While IVF offers hope, it does not circumvent the biological clock entirely; it simply provides an additional pathway for those facing fertility struggles.

## Egg Freezing as Fertility Insurance

Egg freezing, or oocyte cryopreservation, is another option growing in popularity, particularly among women who want to delay motherhood. The procedure allows women to preserve eggs at a younger age, theoretically providing them with better-quality eggs should they choose to conceive later in life. But while egg freezing can extend the reproductive window, it is not a foolproof solution. The success of future pregnancies depends on the number and quality of eggs frozen, as well as the woman's health when she attempts pregnancy. On average, only a fraction of frozen eggs will successfully fertilize, implant, and result in a live birth.

Moreover, freezing eggs at a later age, such as in the late 30s or early 40s, may offer limited advantages since age-related decline in egg quality remains a factor. The technology holds promise but cannot wholly suspend or bypass the natural decline in fertility.

## "Healthy Lifestyle" as a Cure-All

Another misconception is that a healthy lifestyle—exercise, balanced nutrition, stress management—can stave off fertility decline. While maintaining overall health can positively impact reproductive health, it cannot override the biological limits on egg quality and supply. Women's reproductive organs are sensitive to age, and lifestyle adjustments alone cannot change the number of eggs a woman is born with or the rate at which they age.

## The Reality Check: Embracing Knowledge and Options

Understanding the biological timeline of fertility is a step toward informed and proactive decision-making. While society's narrative often emphasizes personal agency and independence, biology demands its own consideration. Fertility treatments and lifestyle choices are invaluable parts of modern reproductive planning, but they are complements to—not substitutes for—the body's natural cycles.

The goal is not to instill fear but to promote awareness. Knowing the truth about fertility timelines and dispelling myths around modern reproductive technologies empowers women to make choices that are right for their lives, not based on assumptions or misinformation. Knowledge of one's fertility potential, when paired with the realities of biology and the limitations of science, opens the door to a more intentional, empowered approach to family planning.

# CHAPTER 3

## THE IMPORTANCE OF FERTILITY PRESERVATION

As women today navigate careers, relationships, and self-discovery, the concept of fertility preservation has become a valuable tool for those who may want to extend their reproductive timelines. Fertility preservation is not just about "buying time"; it's about empowerment, giving women an option to align their reproductive goals with personal and professional aspirations. But while the technology behind egg freezing and fertility preservation is increasingly accessible, it remains under-discussed, leaving many women without the knowledge they need to make informed decisions. In this chapter, we'll explore what fertility preservation truly entails, why early education is critical, and the financial and ethical dimensions that shape this choice.

## Egg Freezing and Fertility Preservation: Taking Control of Reproductive Futures

Egg freezing, technically known as oocyte cryopreservation, has gained prominence as a way for women to preserve fertility potential, providing a "snapshot" of their reproductive health at a younger age. By freezing eggs when they are most viable—typically in the late 20s or early 30s—women may reduce the pressure of trying to conceive naturally at a later age when egg quality is likely to have declined.

The process itself is complex but rooted in a straightforward principle: by harvesting and freezing eggs during a woman's peak reproductive years, it's possible to use those eggs in the future when natural fertility might otherwise have diminished. After undergoing a series of hormone injections to stimulate egg production, a woman undergoes an egg retrieval procedure where mature eggs are collected, frozen, and stored until they are needed. When the time comes, the frozen eggs can be thawed, fertilized through IVF, and implanted into the uterus to attempt pregnancy.

Egg freezing doesn't guarantee future pregnancy success, but it offers a measure of control that previous generations lacked. For women who know they may want children but aren't ready due to personal, professional, or financial reasons, fertility preservation offers a path forward—a chance to pursue motherhood on their own terms. The science may not be infallible, but it does provide an option in the face of a biological clock that often feels unrelenting.

## Why This Needs to Be Discussed More: Raising Public Awareness

Despite its potential, fertility preservation is still a topic that often goes undiscussed. Many women remain unaware of egg freezing until they reach an age where natural fertility has already begun to decline. The lack of information and resources can leave women feeling blindsided by their own biology, caught off guard by the realities of fertility decline.

Research has shown that many women regret not having considered egg freezing earlier. In a 2018 study published in Human Reproduction, women who froze their eggs reported that they wished they had been given more information about fertility decline and options for preservation at a younger age. This regret underscores the need for public awareness and early education on fertility health—both for women and men.

Increasing awareness isn't just about promoting egg freezing; it's about empowering individuals to make proactive choices about their reproductive futures. Fertility discussions, once confined to doctors' offices or private conversations, should be part of broader health education. By normalizing conversations about fertility, we give people the information needed to make informed choices, whether they pursue egg freezing or simply plan their lives with a clearer understanding of their biological timelines.

In addition, fostering a culture of openness around fertility preservation may help to dismantle stigmas associated with it. Egg freezing is sometimes seen as a "last resort," an option for those who haven't "settled down" or "found the right partner." But this perspective is outdated and dismissive of the nuanced realities modern women face. Egg freezing isn't a signal of personal failure—it's a proactive, empowering choice that reflects women's agency over their lives and futures.

**Financial and Ethical Considerations: The Costs and Concerns of Fertility Preservation**

While fertility preservation holds promise, it is not without financial and ethical challenges that deserve thoughtful consideration. For many, the high costs of egg freezing remain a barrier. In the United States, the cost of a single egg-freezing cycle ranges from $6,000 to $15,000, with additional expenses for hormone medications and annual storage fees. Because multiple cycles may be needed to freeze a sufficient number of eggs, the total cost can be substantial, reaching upwards of $20,000 to $30,000. Similarly, in Nigeria, Fertility preservation/IVF treatment can cost N2,800,000 and above with additional cost of N1,300,000 and above for drugs. Annual storage renewal for egg freezing is about N375,000.

For many women, especially those from lower socioeconomic backgrounds, this cost makes fertility preservation out of reach. Insurance coverage for egg freezing is limited, often restricted to medical cases like cancer where treatments may threaten fertility. This disparity in access raises important ethical questions about who can afford the luxury of reproductive choice. If egg freezing is to be considered a valid option for women's health, there's an argument to be made for more inclusive policies that make it accessible to a broader population.

Some companies have begun offering egg freezing as an employee benefit, framing it as a means to support women's career aspirations and alleviate the pressure of balancing work with family planning. However, these corporate-sponsored programs raise additional ethical considerations. While they appear to offer women greater freedom, critics argue that they subtly incentivize women to delay childbearing to prioritize their careers, potentially leading to pressures that shape reproductive decisions in ways that benefit corporations rather than individuals.

Beyond financial concerns, there are ethical questions surrounding the concept of "preserving" fertility itself. Does egg freezing create unrealistic expectations? For some, the ability to freeze eggs can bring false assurances that pregnancy will happen whenever they choose. As we've explored in previous chapters, fertility preservation is not a guarantee of future success. While egg freezing offers a chance, it doesn't eliminate the complexities of conception, pregnancy, or even parenting later in life.

Moreover, there are cultural and societal implications to consider. Fertility preservation represents a shift in how we view family planning, relationships, and reproductive health. Are we moving toward a society that values career over family or one that offers women true autonomy? Do we risk commodifying fertility, turning reproduction into a matter of finance and planning rather than an experience of life's natural rhythms? These questions don't have easy answers, but they are important considerations for anyone thinking about the broader implications of fertility preservation.

## Charting a Future of Empowered Choice

The choice to freeze one's eggs is deeply personal, shaped by unique life circumstances, values, and aspirations. It's a choice that must balance the realities of biology, the possibilities of science, and the limitations of our current understanding of reproductive health. Fertility preservation offers hope for those who want more control over their reproductive futures, but it also calls for a measured, realistic perspective.

For many, fertility preservation is about reclaiming agency in a world that is rapidly changing. It is a step toward aligning one's family dreams with the complexities of modern life. However, as with any significant choice, it is essential to enter this journey with both optimism and awareness, embracing the opportunities it presents while remaining grounded in the realities that shape it.

As we move forward, we must work to make information about fertility preservation accessible and destigmatized, ensuring that women can approach this choice with clarity, confidence, and support. Whether a woman chooses to preserve her fertility or not, what matters is that she has the knowledge and opportunity to decide on her own terms. In a world that sometimes limits women's choices, fertility preservation is a chance for freedom—and a future shaped by empowered decisions.

# CHAPTER 4

## SOCIETAL NORMS HOLDING WOMEN BACK

As much as modern women have gained autonomy over their choices, society's expectations around marriage, motherhood, and family persist as powerful forces that shape life paths, often in subtle and unseen ways. Cultural pressures remain ingrained in the social fabric, affecting how women view their own desires, decisions, and possibilities. Different circumstances influence the reasons a woman might choose single motherhood: aging fertility, failed relationships, unsuitable/unavailable life partners, personal autonomy, and a powerful desire to raise a child.

This chapter examines societal norms, exploring how they shape the lives of women and why challenging them is critical to achieving true autonomy.

## Cultural Pressures: The Weight of Societal Expectations

Society's expectations for women to marry and bear children, while less overt than in previous generations, remain embedded in cultural messages, familial expectations, and even workplace dynamics. From a young age, women are often socialized to see family and motherhood as an inevitable life milestone, something "good" women aspire to achieve. As they move into adulthood, these expectations become more pronounced, transforming into pressures that influence not only how women view their futures but also how they are perceived by others.

The result is a culture that often values women based on their marital and maternal status. A woman who chooses to focus on her career, who remains single, or who delays childbearing may be met with subtle judgments or well-meaning questions that imply her life is somehow "missing" something. Family gatherings, social events, and even casual conversations often carry the weight of unspoken assumptions about a woman's role, reinforcing the idea that happiness and fulfillment are found through partnership and motherhood.

For women who may want to explore their careers, enjoy personal freedom, or simply aren't ready for marriage and children, these pressures can feel limiting and isolating. The societal narrative remains: a woman's worth and success are inextricably tied to her ability to marry and become a mother. This message not only influences individual women but reinforces a culture that still views single or child-free women as anomalies or as women who are somehow "delayed" in reaching the expected milestones of adult life.

## The Fear of Judgment: Choosing Motherhood Outside of Marriage

Choosing to parent outside of a traditional partnership structure often triggers questions about a woman's competence, her child's well-being, and her commitment to family values—all because her path doesn't conform to conventional standards.

This fear of judgment is amplified by deeply ingrained beliefs about the ideal family structure. Societal messages frequently reinforce the notion that a "complete" family consists of two parents—a mother and a father—suggesting that anything else is a deviation from what is best for the child. This perspective overlooks the diverse ways families thrive and the strength of a woman's desire to create a loving, stable environment for her child, regardless of her marital status.

Nevertheless, the fear of judgment often compels many women to put off the decision to have children until they find a suitable partner, sometimes indefinitely, despite a strong desire for motherhood.

This reluctance to pursue motherhood alone, fueled by the potential for social scrutiny, reflects society's need to expand its definitions of family and success. A woman's choice to raise a child should be celebrated as a testament to her agency, her commitment, and her love, rather than questioned based on outdated social expectations.

## Stigma of Single Motherhood

In a world that has made strides toward inclusivity and diversity, single motherhood remains a topic shrouded in stigma, often unspoken yet deeply felt. Women who choose to raise children on their own are frequently subject to judgment, from whispered remarks to overt criticisms.

The stigma of single motherhood often stems from assumptions about a woman's motivations, values, and even her perceived ability to provide a "complete" upbringing for her child. She may be judged as "selfish" for choosing motherhood without a traditional family structure, or as "irresponsible" for supposedly putting her child at a disadvantage. Unfortunately, the stigma can extend to the workplace and social circles, where women who become mothers on their own may face assumptions about their motivations, finances, or ability to balance work and parenting.

The general misconception that a single mother lacks the resources or capacity to raise a well-adjusted child prevails. This viewpoint is not only outdated but fails to consider the resilience, planning, and resourcefulness required to take on single parenthood. In many cases, single mothers have carefully evaluated their circumstances, built strong support networks, and made informed decisions about their futures.

## Personal Stories: Women Who Defied Societal Expectations

These stories are not just accounts of resilience; they are narratives of courage, intention, and empowerment.

Consider the story of Dana, a woman in her late 30s who always envisioned herself as a mother but never felt pressured to marry. After years of dating without finding a partner who aligned with her life goals, Dana decided to pursue motherhood independently. With a stable career and a close-knit network of friends and family, she knew she could provide a loving home for a child. Despite facing questions about her decision from coworkers, friends, and even family members, Dana held firm. She opted for IVF with a sperm donor and today, she is the proud mother of a young daughter and an advocate for women considering solo parenthood. Her journey wasn't without challenges, but it has filled her life with purpose and joy.

Another story comes from Kemi, a woman who chose to adopt as a single parent. Her family and friends were initially supportive of her choice to adopt, but many questioned her ability to "do it alone" as she began navigating the adoption process. Kemi knew, however, that she had a strong desire to parent, a good support system, and a heart full of love to give. As she awaited the arrival of her adopted son, Kemi prepared meticulously, creating a home that would meet his needs and surround him with stability and love. Today, she reflects on the journey with pride, seeing herself as part of a broader movement redefining what it means to be a family.

There is also Aliyah, 28, a researcher who got a scholarship for her Ph.D. program in a top ivy league school in the UK. She discussed with her fiancé, and both agreed they were not ready to get married or have children due to their demanding professions. She decided to freeze her eggs before departing for her studies which may take her 4 years to complete.

These women and countless others reveal the multifaceted realities of women's fertility journeys. Their paths are unique, their reasons varied, but what they share is a commitment to redefining motherhood on their terms. By telling their stories, we break down stereotypes and illuminate the depth of love and resilience that underpins single motherhood.

## Breaking Free from Social Norms: Redefining the Timeline of Womanhood

If we are to foster a culture where women feel empowered to make their own reproductive choices, we must challenge the restrictive norms that hold them back. At the heart of this movement is the recognition that a woman's timeline is her own and that "normal" no longer means one-size-fits-all. By breaking down these cultural expectations, we open up space for women to pursue marriage and motherhood on terms that feel authentic and fulfilling to them—not dictated by societal pressures.

The concept of "normalcy" has long been a barrier to women's autonomy. Whether it's the age by which women are expected to marry, the ideal family structure, or the narrative that happiness is found through traditional pathways, these norms subtly limit women's choices. For many, the desire to fit in, to belong, or to be viewed as "successful" in the eyes of society can lead to decisions that feel rushed or misaligned with personal aspirations. Reclaiming ownership over these life choices is a matter of giving women the freedom to define their paths without feeling inadequate, judged, or misunderstood.

One of the most empowering ways to break free from these expectations is through open conversation. Talking openly about the diverse paths women take allows society to witness the myriad ways in which happiness, fulfillment, and family can manifest. When we celebrate women who choose non-traditional paths—whether that means delaying marriage, having children on their own, or opting not to have children at all—we send a message that success and joy are not confined to one formula.

Education and awareness also play a pivotal role in challenging norms. For young women, early exposure to ideas about career options, personal growth, and reproductive choices provides the foundation for making informed, empowered decisions later in life. When we educate girls and young women about their options and encourage them to explore various life paths without fear of judgment, we lay the groundwork for a society where individual autonomy is valued above outdated cultural scripts.

## Redefining Autonomy for the Next Generation

Ultimately, the push to redefine societal norms around marriage and motherhood isn't just about giving women the freedom to choose their own timelines; it's about building a culture that respects and values those choices. By creating a world where women feel free to make decisions based on their dreams and desires—not on the judgments of others—we foster a society that embraces diversity, supports autonomy, and allows each person to live a life that feels true to who they are.

Challenging these norms is no small feat. It requires collective efforts to dismantle stereotypes, broaden societal definitions of family, and celebrate the diverse experiences that make up the fabric of modern womanhood. But it is a challenge worth taking on. When we champion the right of every woman to decide when and how to pursue marriage or motherhood, we open doors to a future where each life path is met with acceptance, curiosity, and respect.

The journey toward autonomy in the face of societal expectations is deeply personal, but it is also profoundly collective. As more women challenge these norms, they contribute to a broader shift—one where every choice is validated, where independence is respected, and where family is defined not by convention, but by love, commitment, and intentionality.

# CHAPTER 5

## MEN AS PARTNERS FOR WOMEN'S FERTILITY

When it comes to fertility and reproductive rights, the role of men is often viewed from the sidelines, as if these issues are solely a "woman's problem." However, the reality is far more complex. Men play a dual role: as both influencers of women's reproductive choices—sometimes in ways that hinder progress—and as indispensable partners in fostering supportive environments for fertility and reproductive health.

This chapter delves into the ways men, through societal structures, behaviors, and choices, can act as both perpetrators of systemic barriers and as allies in the journey toward fertility empowerment and reproductive rights.

### The Role of Patriarchy and Toxic Masculinity

Patriarchy has long shaped societal norms surrounding fertility, often placing the burden of reproduction squarely on women while absolving men of accountability. This imbalance is exacerbated by toxic masculinity, which enforces rigid gender roles and stigmatizes vulnerability. Together, these forces create environments where women face additional pressures and limitations in exercising their reproductive rights.

1. **Patriarchy's Influence on Reproductive Decisions**
   In many cultures, men hold decision-making power within relationships and families. Women may face coercion to conform to male-dominated timelines or expectations, such as delaying motherhood to align with a partner's readiness or prioritizing a man's career over their own biological clock. When long term relationships (5 to 10 years) which was promising to result in marriage ends abruptly, the woman's fertility aspiration is often adversely affected.

2. **Stigma Around Male Infertility**
   Male infertility accounts for nearly half of infertility cases, yet the topic is rarely discussed. Toxic masculinity perpetuates the belief that fertility issues are a sign of weakness, forcing

many men to avoid testing or treatment. This stigma shifts the focus—and blame—onto women, often delaying diagnoses and solutions.

3. **Control Over Contraception and Fertility Preservation** Men's attitudes toward contraception and fertility preservation also play a significant role. In relationships where men discourage or control access to birth control, women are left without autonomy over their reproductive health. Similarly, a lack of male support for fertility preservation measures, such as egg freezing, especially when the man controls the financial resources, can hinder women from making proactive choices.

## Men as Partners: Supporting Women Through Fertility Journeys

For true gender equity in reproductive health, men must move beyond traditional roles and become active, empathetic partners in fertility journeys. Here are key areas where men can make a positive impact:

1. **Shared Accountability** Fertility is a shared responsibility, and

men must be proactive in their own reproductive health. This includes undergoing semen analysis, addressing lifestyle factors that impact fertility, and being open to discussing potential male-factor infertility.

2. **Emotional Support**
Fertility challenges can take a significant emotional toll on women. Men can provide meaningful support by:

- Actively participating in discussions about fertility treatments or family planning.
- Attending medical appointments and being informed about procedures.
- Offering reassurance and understanding during moments of frustration or grief.

3. **Challenging Societal Norms**
Men can help dismantle patriarchal norms by normalizing conversations about infertility and reproductive health. Sharing personal stories, supporting open dialogue, and advocating for gender equity in fertility decision-making are critical steps that

can enhance an enabling environment for women's fertility decisions.

**Practical Actions for Men to Foster Supportive Partnerships**

To be effective partners in fertility journeys, men need to embrace specific attitudes and actions:

- **Educate Themselves**: Gain a clear understanding of fertility, including male-factor infertility, and how reproductive health affects both partners.
- **Be Present**: Actively engage in discussions about reproductive plans, treatments, and options. Show up—physically and emotionally—during challenging times.
- **Adopt Healthy Habits**: Support reproductive health by addressing lifestyle factors like diet, exercise, and avoiding harmful substances such as tobacco and excessive alcohol.
- **Encourage Autonomy**: Respect and support a woman's right to make decisions about her own body, whether that's pursuing treatments, delaying

motherhood, or considering alternative paths to parenthood.

- **Advocate for Change**: Use their voices to challenge societal norms and push for policies that promote equitable access to fertility education and care for women and men.

## The Road Ahead: Building Collaborative Futures

Men have the power to be transformative allies in the journey toward reproductive empowerment. By addressing the negative impacts of patriarchy and toxic masculinity, while stepping into supportive and accountable roles, men can help create environments where women feel empowered to make timely, informed reproductive choices.

True progress requires men to reframe their roles—not just as passive participants but as active, empathetic partners. Together, both men and women can dismantle barriers, foster healthier relationships, and build a future where fertility decisions are collaborative and empowering.

# CHAPTER 6

# THE INFLUENCE OF RELIGION ON FERTILITY CHOICES

Religion is one of the most powerful forces shaping individual decisions and societal attitudes toward fertility. They influence how women and men perceive parenthood, fertility preservation, single motherhood, and assisted reproductive technologies (ART). While these influences can offer support and guidance, they can also perpetuate stigmas, restrict autonomy, and hinder timely reproductive decisions.

This chapter explores how religious and cultural beliefs—particularly in Christianity and Islam—affect fertility choices, examining perspectives from both developed and developing countries.

## Christianity and Fertility Choices

Christianity's stance on fertility varies widely across denominations and cultural contexts, often shaped by interpretations of scripture and church teachings.

1. **Fertility Preservation**:

   - **Supportive Perspectives**: In many Christian communities, fertility preservation (e.g., egg or sperm freezing) is increasingly accepted, particularly when aligned with marital goals. For example, couples may choose fertility preservation to ensure they can have children after overcoming health challenges, such as cancer.
   - **Ethical Concerns**: Some conservative Christian groups raise concerns about freezing embryos, as they consider embryos to hold moral status. These groups advocate for the use of technologies that align with their pro-life principles, such as freezing eggs rather than embryos.

2. **Single Motherhood**:

   - **Cultural Stigma**: In many Christian communities, single motherhood outside marriage is often stigmatized. This is particularly pronounced in conservative settings where traditional family structures are emphasized.

- **Shifting Attitudes**: However, in developed countries, many liberal Christian groups are embracing single motherhood, viewing it as a personal choice rather than a moral failing. Support systems like church-based childcare programs for single mothers are becoming more common.

3. **Assisted Reproductive Technologies (ART)**:

- **Acceptance**: Some Christian denominations, particularly in developed countries, accept ART as a means of fulfilling the biblical mandate to "be fruitful and multiply." However, they may encourage the use of techniques that avoid creating excess embryos.
- **Resistance**: More conservative factions, especially in developing countries, often

reject ART, citing concerns about playing God, manipulating natural processes, or the potential destruction of embryos.

## Islam and Fertility Choices

Islamic teachings on fertility are rooted in the Quran and Hadith, with scholars offering diverse interpretations based on cultural and contextual factors.

1. **Fertility Preservation**:

    - **Permissibility**: Many Islamic scholars permit fertility preservation within the context of marriage, especially in cases where health conditions threaten fertility. Egg and sperm freezing are generally accepted as long as the materials are used exclusively between the husband and wife.
    - **Cultural Hesitation**: In conservative Muslim communities, especially in developing countries, fertility preservation is sometimes viewed with suspicion due to

limited awareness and fears of cultural taboo.

2.  **Single Motherhood**:

- **Cultural and Religious Resistance**: In Islam, traditional family structures are highly valued, and single motherhood outside marriage is generally discouraged. Single mothers often face significant stigma, particularly in conservative Muslim-majority countries, where cultural norms reinforce the importance of marriage.
- **Emerging Acceptance**: In developed countries, where Muslim communities are increasingly exposed to diverse family structures, single motherhood through ART or adoption is slowly gaining acceptance among progressive groups.

3.  **Assisted Reproductive Technologies (ART)**:

- **Permissibility Within Marriage**: ART is widely accepted in Islam when used within the confines of marriage. Techniques such as IVF are permitted as long as they involve the husband and wife's genetic material.
- **Donor Material and Surrogacy**: The use of donor eggs, sperm, or surrogacy is often prohibited in Islamic law, as it is seen as violating the sanctity of marriage and lineage. However, attitudes are evolving in some developed Muslim-majority countries, where reproductive technologies are being reinterpreted to align with modern needs.

## Practical Steps Toward Inclusivity

1.  **Education and Dialogue**:
Religious and cultural leaders should foster open conversations about fertility choices, emphasizing compassion and

understanding rather than judgment. Consultations with single women (and men) who desire to be parents should be convened to understand their needs, challenges and provide the required social and spiritual support.

2. **Policy Reform**:
   Faith Institutions should develop clear policies on to make fertility education part of their pre-marital classes. Matured singles who wish to become parents should also be supported and encouraged to explore the most suitable fertility pathway for them in accordance with the teachings of their faith. Religious institutions should also work with Government to create policies that make fertility treatments accessible and affordable.

3. **Healthcare Integration**:
   Healthcare providers working on facilities owned by religious institutions should be trained and equipped to offer comprehensive reproductive health services tailored to diverse populations.

4.  **Celebrate all Children**:
    Children born or adopted by single
    mothers should receive the same
    recognition as children born by couples
    to discourage discrimination.

## Final Thoughts

As the population of single women who desire
to have children is growing across diverse
cultures, religious and traditional leaders are
obligated to reflect, consult and provide clear
guidance on their institutional position on
single parenthood.

By fostering inclusive dialogue, challenging
outdated norms, and creating supportive
systems, religious institutions can create a
safe space for single women to make
reproductive choices that align with their faith
and personal values, free from judgment and
barriers.

Through collaboration between religious
leaders, cultural influencers, and reproductive
health advocates, we can ensure that every
woman—regardless of her background—has
the opportunity to make informed decisions
about her fertility and family-building
journey.

# CHAPTER 7

## THE ROLE OF POLICY AND ADVOCACY

Women's reproductive choices and their ability to manage their fertility in a society that increasingly delays motherhood isn't solely a personal issue. It's also a public matter that calls for systemic support, encompassing government policy, employer benefits, healthcare access, and public education. While individual choices are essential, these decisions exist within a larger structure that can either empower or hinder women in pursuing their desired life paths. This chapter explores the pressing need for policy reform and advocacy efforts aimed at supporting modern women, from workplace benefits to public education initiatives on fertility and reproductive health.

# A Call for Change: Challenging the Status Quo

In a world where marriage and motherhood increasingly occur later in life, it's imperative to cultivate an environment that respects and supports individual journeys, allowing women the freedom to decide how, when, and if they wish to navigate their fertility.

Challenging the status quo requires a holistic, collaborative effort from every sector of society. It's not enough to simply raise awareness; we must drive systemic change that creates a culture of empowerment, equity, and education. Below, we explore practical and proactive ways that key stakeholders can foster change to support the future of fertility and womanhood.

## 1. The Role of Policymakers

Policymakers hold the power to enact structural reforms that make reproductive healthcare accessible, affordable, and equitable.

The high cost of procedures like egg freezing, in-vitro fertilization (IVF), and comprehensive fertility testing creates a barrier for many women. Public policy has yet to fully address this gap, leaving women to navigate a healthcare system that often treats fertility as a luxury rather than a central aspect of health and well-being. Addressing these challenges requires policy shifts at multiple levels, from expanding healthcare coverage to implementing workplace benefits that support reproductive autonomy.

- **Expand Access to Fertility Treatments**: Create subsidies, tax breaks, or insurance mandates that cover fertility treatments and preservation options, ensuring that financial barriers don't prevent women from accessing care.
- **Promote Comprehensive Reproductive Health Legislation**: Enact policies that mandate fertility education in schools, regulate the use of reproductive technologies, and protect the rights of women to make autonomous choices about their fertility. As recommended by WHO, approve incorporating fertility education into existing Comprehensive Sexuality Education curriculums.

- **Improve Adoption and Foster Care Policies:** ensure processes for adoption are transparent, accessible and inclusive of eligible single women (and men).
- **Parental Leave and Family Policies**: Design inclusive parental leave policies that support diverse family structures and encourage shared parenting responsibilities.

## 2. The Role of Educators

Education is the cornerstone of empowerment, and fertility education must start as early as high school and continue through college and professional life to ensure that women and men are equipped to make informed decisions about their reproductive futures. This information is also vital for young women making decisions that affect their futures, from career paths to family planning.

- **Provide Fertility Education in Schools**: Teach students about fertility timelines, reproductive health, and the impact of lifestyle choices on fertility from a young age.

- **Destigmatize Reproductive Health Conversations**: Create a safe, inclusive environment in schools and universities where discussions about fertility, family planning, and reproductive challenges are normalized.
- **Promote Lifelong Learning**: Offer community workshops, online resources, and public campaigns that provide ongoing education about fertility and reproductive rights.

## 3. The Role of Healthcare Providers

Healthcare professionals are pivotal in guiding individuals through their reproductive health journeys.

- **Enhance Training for Reproductive Health Specialists**: Ensure that doctors, nurses, and counselors are well-equipped to discuss fertility preservation, treatment options, and the emotional impact of reproductive challenges.

- **Advocate for Early Screenings and Preventive Care**: Encourage routine fertility assessments and screenings for conditions like endometriosis or PCOS, empowering women to take proactive steps. Client counselling on age-related fertility for women under 35 should be provided.
- **Provide Compassionate and Inclusive Care**: Develop patient-centered approaches that respect cultural sensitivities, gender identities, and diverse family-building goals.

## 4. The Role of Employers

Workplaces play a critical role in shaping how women balance their careers with their reproductive choices. For many women, the workplace is more than a place to earn a living; it's an environment that shapes long-term life decisions, including the choice of when and how to become a parent. Access to fertility preservation through health insurance could be a game-changer, allowing women to consider their reproductive choices without the pressure of financial burden.

- **Offer Fertility Benefits**: Provide employee health insurance plans that include coverage for fertility treatments, egg freezing, and other reproductive health services.
- **Foster Work-Life Balance**: Implement flexible work schedules, remote work options, and parental leave policies that accommodate the needs of working parents and caregivers.
- **Support Awareness Campaigns**: Partner with reproductive health organizations to educate employees about fertility and encourage open dialogue.

## 5. The Role of Community Members

Communities have the power to normalize conversations about fertility and support individuals navigating reproductive challenges.

- **Create Support Networks**: Establish local groups or online forums where individuals can share experiences, resources, and emotional support.

- **Challenge Stigmas**: Actively counter myths, taboos, and judgmental attitudes surrounding infertility, single motherhood, and assisted reproductive technologies.
- **Engage Men as Allies**: Encourage men to participate in reproductive health conversations, recognizing that fertility and parenting are shared responsibilities.

## 6. The Role of Religious Institutions

Religious and cultural organizations wield significant influence over societal norms and individual decisions.

- **Promote Compassionate Messaging**: Encourage clergy and religious leaders to address reproductive health with empathy, supporting women's choices rather than perpetuating stigma.
- **Foster Inclusive Discussions**: Open channels for dialogue that consider the intersection of faith, fertility, and modern reproductive technologies.
- **Support Community-Based Initiatives**: Partner with healthcare providers and policymakers to offer

resources and support for individuals facing fertility challenges.

## Moving Toward a Future of Empowered Choice

The role of policy and advocacy in supporting women's reproductive choices cannot be overstated. Systemic change creates an environment where women feel supported in pursuing their aspirations, balancing careers, and making informed family decisions without fear of social or financial penalties. By addressing fertility as a central part of healthcare, advocating for workplace fertility benefits, and promoting fertility education, we build a society that values and empowers every woman's right to choose her own path.

Reform doesn't happen overnight, but progress is possible when policies reflect the lives and realities of those they are meant to serve. In a society where the timeline of motherhood is increasingly flexible, supporting women in their reproductive choices is both a matter of equality and a commitment to fostering a more inclusive and supportive world.

When women are empowered with knowledge, resources, and options, they gain not just the ability to navigate their own fertility but the freedom to make choices that reflect their truest values and aspirations. This is the power of policy and advocacy—to create a world where each woman's path is respected, supported, and celebrated, enabling her to shape her life on her own terms.

# CHAPTER 8

## THE FUTURE OF FERTILITY AND WOMANHOOD

As we close this exploration of fertility in a rapidly changing world, it becomes increasingly clear that we stand at a pivotal moment in our understanding of womanhood and reproductive choices. The dialogue surrounding fertility is evolving, yet the need for meaningful change is urgent. It's time to challenge the status quo, dismantle outdated norms, and create space for more inclusive and empowering perspectives on women's fertility.

### Empowering Women to Take Action

To all the women reading this book, remember that your fertility journey is yours to navigate. You possess the power to shape your reproductive future through informed decision-making and proactive engagement with your health. Educate yourself about your body, the options available to you, and the implications of your choices.

Conduct a fertility assessment to know your reproductive status and treat any medical conditions that may affect your fertility promptly.

Your fertility journey should be treated as an integral part of your life plans in recognition of your limited biological fertility window. Remaining in a long-term relationship with no plan and commitment for marriage and parenthood may jeopardize your chances of having children later. Be intentional about your relationships and have open and timely communication with your partner about your fertility goals and desires to foster shared values and synergy.

If you are still single by age 30, be proactive to consider freezing your eggs if it is affordable and accessible to you. Seek a credible fertility specialist for consultation and assessment.

Embracing your power also means rejecting the fear or stigma that may accompany your fertility decisions. The more women speak openly about their experiences—whether it's about delaying motherhood, pursuing fertility treatments, or choosing single motherhood—the more we normalize these narratives. By sharing your story, you can inspire others and contribute to a collective movement that celebrates women's autonomy and diversity in reproductive choices.

## Proactive Steps for Fertility Education

One of the most powerful tools in a woman's reproductive toolkit is knowledge. Understanding how fertility works, including the biological clock, the implications of aging on fertility, and the options available for fertility preservation, can make all the difference in planning for the future. Often, women are either underinformed or receive critical information too late to act effectively. By equipping women with comprehensive, science-backed knowledge about their bodies, we provide them with the agency to make empowered choices.

For instance, early awareness of fertility preservation options—such as egg freezing, embryo freezing, or IVF—enables women to consider these possibilities long before age may affect success rates. However, it's also essential for women to recognize that while science offers valuable tools, there are no absolute guarantees. Fertility preservation can be an effective part of reproductive planning, but it's important to approach these options with realistic expectations. Being informed means making choices from a place of understanding rather than urgency.

Moreover, educating oneself about fertility is not limited to understanding technology. It also means recognizing the significance of lifestyle factors that can impact reproductive health. Nutrition, stress management, sleep, and physical activity all contribute to overall well-being, which in turn can influence fertility. Understanding these factors and making intentional lifestyle choices can support a healthy reproductive system and empower women to approach fertility as a part of overall health, not a separate or secondary concern.

## The Importance of Building Support Networks for the Fertility Journey

While individual knowledge is critical, no woman should have to navigate her fertility journey alone. Support networks—whether through family, friends, or specialized communities—play a crucial role in offering guidance, emotional support, and a sense of solidarity. These networks can be especially valuable for women who face stigma or misunderstanding from their immediate circles. A strong support system provides a safe space for open conversations about fertility, including challenges, choices, and the emotional complexities that often accompany them.

In recent years, many online and in-person communities have emerged, offering platforms for women to share their experiences, exchange resources, and offer mutual encouragement. These groups vary in focus, from fertility preservation and IVF support groups to communities for single mothers by choice. They provide a wealth of shared knowledge, affirming that no one is alone in facing these questions and decisions. This collective wisdom can help demystify the fertility journey and remind women that their experiences are shared and understood by others.

Professional support can also be part of a woman's network, including reproductive endocrinologists, therapists, fertility counselors, and nutritionists specializing in reproductive health. A multidisciplinary approach can provide well-rounded support, addressing the emotional, physical, and medical aspects of the fertility journey. For example, fertility counselors can help women manage the emotional side of fertility preservation, while reproductive endocrinologists offer insights into the most effective fertility options based on individual circumstances. These experts not only provide professional guidance but also help women feel supported in their choices, reinforcing their agency and confidence.

## Redefining Societal Expectations Around Fertility

Beyond personal choices and individual journeys, societal expectations around fertility profoundly influence how women experience and approach motherhood. For too long, the social narrative has emphasized early marriage and motherhood as markers of "success," implicitly questioning the paths of women who choose to delay or redefine these milestones. This narrative need reshaping to celebrate all reproductive choices equally—whether a woman chooses early motherhood, fertility preservation, adoption, or even deciding to remain child-free.

Shaping a new narrative means shifting the dialogue from what women "should" do to how women can be supported in what they choose to do. By challenging stereotypes and outdated norms, we create space for each woman to define her reproductive choices on her terms. We can also encourage society to view fertility not as a countdown clock or a race but as a personal decision that deserves respect, understanding, and support.

Educational campaigns, media representation, and public advocacy can help create a culture where fertility choices are viewed through a lens of respect and autonomy. Television, books, and social media can play a powerful role in normalizing diverse family structures and fertility decisions. Stories about women pursuing fertility preservation, choosing single motherhood, or balancing career and family contribute to a broader, more inclusive view of womanhood and parenthood.

## Final Thoughts: Building a Supportive Society

As we look toward the future, let us envision a society that fully supports all women—single women, mothers, and those navigating their fertility journeys in myriad ways. This future is not merely aspirational; it is achievable through dedicated efforts to foster a culture of understanding, respect, and inclusivity.

We must work to dismantle the stigma surrounding single motherhood and challenge the cultural pressures that dictate when and how women should become mothers. The narratives we weave today will shape the lives of future generations, allowing young women to embrace their fertility decisions without fear or judgment.

The future of fertility and womanhood lies in our hands. Let us rise to the challenge, champion inclusive perspectives, and ensure that every woman has the opportunity to define her path and pursue her dreams—on her own terms.

The path forward is one of partnership, understanding, and a commitment to honoring each woman's unique vision for her life. Through these efforts, we can truly empower the next generation of women to navigate their fertility journeys with confidence, clarity, and a profound sense of possibility.

# REFERENCES AND FURTHER READING

## Books and Journals

1. American College of Obstetricians and Gynecologists. *Fertility Preservation in Women of Reproductive Age.* ACOG Committee Opinion No. 584. American College of Obstetricians and Gynecologists, 2014.

2. Becker, Gay. *The Elusive Embryo: How Women and Men Approach New Reproductive Technologies.* University of California Press, 2000. *An insightful exploration of the social, cultural, and emotional aspects of fertility preservation and reproductive technologies.*

3. Brody, Jane E. *The Fertility Guide: A Complete Guide to Getting Pregnant and Maximizing Your Chances of Having a Baby.* Wiley, 2001.

4. Greil, Arthur L., et al. "The Experience of Infertility: A Review of Recent Literature." *Sociology of Health & Illness,* vol. 32, no. 1, 2010, pp. 140–

162.

*An academic review discussing the social aspects of infertility and the psychological impact on those who experience it.*

5. Inhorn, Marcia C., and Frank van Balen. *Infertility Around the Globe: New Thinking on Childlessness, Gender, and Reproductive Technologies.* University of California Press, 2002.
*A global perspective on infertility and cultural views on motherhood and family structures.*

6. Petropanagos, Angel. *Reproductive Ethics: New Ideas and Innovations.* Oxford University Press, 2015.
*A book covering the ethical issues surrounding fertility treatments and reproductive choices.*

**Articles and Reports**

7. American Society for Reproductive Medicine. "Age and Fertility: A Guide for Patients." *American Society for*

*Reproductive Medicine,* 2012. *An overview of the biological factors affecting fertility and age-related risks.*

8. Greil, Arthur L., et al. "The Experience of Infertility: A Review of Recent Literature." *Sociology of Health & Illness,* vol. 32, no. 1, 2010, pp. 140–162.

9. Moffitt, Robert A., et al. "Trends in the Fertility Rates of U.S. Women by Education and Income, 1980-2010." *Demography,* vol. 52, no. 4, 2015, pp. 1069–1094.

10. Sobotka, Tomas, and Eva Beaujouan. "Late Motherhood in Low-Fertility Countries: Reproductive Intentions, Trends, and Consequences." *Journal of Biosocial Science,* vol. 50, no. 3, 2018, pp. 386-414.

**Online Resources**

11. Mayo Clinic. "Egg Freezing: A Guide to Fertility Preservation Options." *Mayo Clinic Health System,* 2023. Available at: www.mayoclinic.org

12. Centers for Disease Control and Prevention. "Reproductive Health: Infertility FAQs." *CDC.gov,* 2022. Available at: https://www.cdc.gov/reproductivehealth/infertility/

13. Society for Assisted Reproductive Technology (SART). "Understanding Success Rates for Fertility Treatments." *SART.org,* 2023. Available at: https://www.sart.org/

14. Resolve: The National Infertility Association. "Resources for People Struggling with Infertility." *Resolve.org,* 2023. Available at: https://resolve.org/

## Additional Readings

15. Ellison, Jesse, and Jessica Bennett. *This Is 40 (But Better): Your Guide to Health, Wellness, and Career Fulfillment.* HarperCollins, 2019. *A practical guide to navigating career, fertility, and personal fulfillment in midlife.*

16. Kuperberg, Arielle. "Age at First Birth and the Motherhood Wage Penalty: When Childbearing Delays Pay Off." *Journal of Marriage and Family,* vol. 82, no. 5, 2020, pp. 1595–1613. *A study on the financial impact of delaying motherhood and its effects on women's careers.*

17. Sandelowski, Margarete. *With Child in Mind: Studies of the Personal Encounter with Infertility.* University of Pennsylvania Press, 1993. *An exploration of the emotional dimensions of infertility.*

9 798302 646149